Essential Oils & Weight Loss for Beginners

BY LINDSEY P

Ultimate Guide to Losing Weight, Increasing Energy, Balancing Metabolism & Appetite Using Essential Oils & Aromatherapy

2ND EDITION

Table of Contents

Introduction

I want to thank you and congratulate you for purchasing the book, "Essential Oils & Weight Loss for Beginners".

This book contains proven steps and strategies on how to make essentials oils work for you to help you conquer the battle against the weighing scale and measuring tape by increasing your energy and balancing your metabolism.

It might sound a little far-fetched to hear that certain essential oils can actually help you to fight off your bulges. However, it is indeed possible! By the end of reading this book, you will find yourself more prepared and equipped to make essential oils work to your advantage. Read on to find out how orange peel essential oils can help turn your orange-peeled skin into toned, cellulite-free smooth skin.

Thanks again for purchasing this book, I hope you enjoy it!

Chapter 1: Essential Oils Basics

Before you get to learn which essential oils can help you in weight loss and how these can accomplish that, let us discuss first just what exactly essential oils are.

Essential oils are concentrated liquids that have a tendency to not absorb water. That means it would not mix nor dissolve in water. It also has botanical aroma compounds that will evaporate readily at normal temperature and pressure.

These oils are termed "essential" due to the fact that they contain the very essence of the plants from which they are taken. This also means that they have the specific scent of that plant. Being named as such does not mean that these oils are "essential" or necessary to be healthy. But it is undeniable that they can benefit you in many ways.

The most common process used in extracting these oils is distillation. Lavender, peppermint, and eucalyptus essential oils are the most commonly distilled oils. The different parts of these plants, like the roots, leaves, flowers, and others, are placed inside a distillation apparatus known as an alembic. It is then placed over water and then heated. As the water's temperature rises, it will produce steam that will pass through the part of the plant, which will then vaporize the volatile elements in it. The vaporized compounds will then flow through a cooling coil, which will make it condense and return to a liquid state. The extracted liquid is the pure plant oil that will be collected in a container.

The less common processes include expression, which

involves pressing the plants in a pressing device or machine to squeeze out the oils. Most citrus peels, like orange, lemon, and grapefruit, are expressed to get their essential oils. They can either be pressed mechanically or through a cold-press. The peels of citrus yield a large quantity of oil. Also, producing the fruits is relatively inexpensive. For this reason, essential oils from citrus fruits are less expensive compared to the others.

Another way to get essential oils from plants is by solvent extraction, which involves separating compounds using a funnel that separates the fluids into two different liquids depending on their solubility. Most commonly, flowers undergo this process as they do not have enough volatile compounds for expression. Moreover, the chemical elements of flowers are too delicate and are readily denatured when heated at high temperatures using the process of steam distillation. Therefore, extraction through the use of solvents such as supercritical carbon dioxide is used to get the oils from flowering plants.

Essential oils, also known as plant extracts, are used in cosmetics, soaps, perfumes, food and beverage flavoring. You can find them mixed in most naturally-scented products. Although essential oils are not required for health, these have been applied medically throughout history. They have been used in hair and skin treatments, as cancer cures, in aromatherapy, and many others.

Western and Oriental medicine practitioners often argue about the efficacy of essential oils. Alternative medicine claims essential oils that have curative effects and many can testify to having been directly benefited by these oils. When giving or being given acupressure as well as different kinds of massages, essential oils are used directly on the skin to be absorbed through the pores. They are also diffused by nebulizers and burned as a candle or incense to be absorbed through the lungs.

If you would like to know how certain essential oils can help you to increase your metabolism, boost your energy, and help you lose weight, then please read on to the next chapter.

Chapter 2: How They Work for You

It is absolutely true that using certain essential oils can help you burn fat. However, nothing quite beats the good, old-fashioned proper diet and exercise. Discretion should be used when utilizing essential oils to aid in weight loss. Never should one expect that just essential oils are enough to keep your body fit and trimmed while you overeat and under-exercise.

That being said though, essential oils coupled with proper diet and exercise can do wonders for your body. After all, losing weight is not just about what you eat and do. It is also about how you feel about your body and self.

Certain essential oils can help you when you are overeating during certain events or experiences in your life. Let's face it: we eat our feelings every now and then. Whenever we are sorely distressed over something, we will almost instantly head to our favorite restaurant or food stall to eat that devilishly delicious, decadent chocolate cake or some hot, crispy deep fried poultry and root crops. Whichever the case, essential oils can give you comfort from the things you are going through. Otherwise, they only would have made you eat non-stop.

The ability to directly burn fat tissue is not a property that can be found in any single essential oil. Instead, there are many that can help boost your metabolism. The better your metabolism, the faster you can trim through fat deposits in your body, thus assisting in your goal to lose weight. Choosing a good essential oil that enhances your metabolism and boosts your energy will be a great addition to your aromatherapy arsenal.

Many citrus fruit essential oils have this metabolism-balancing and energy boosting properties. This family includes lemons, bergamot, grapefruits, and oranges. Other than these, you can also find the same properties in herb oils like basil, sandalwood and rosemary. Spice essential oils like those from peppermint, ginger, and cinnamon also have these abovementioned features.

There are many different ways in which you can mix and use these essential oils to your benefit depending on what you need them for. In the next chapter, we will talk about the essential oils taken from citrus fruits.

Chapter 3: Citrus Essential Oils

It has long been proven by scientists that there is a strong link between what you smell, how you feel, and the eating pattern that you have. Often, we take our senses for granted, not realizing just how strongly it affects our brain and behavior. You would agree that there is more than one time when your stomach grumbles like it is hungry when in fact you just ate a short while. It is your appetite talking. Steadily inhaling citrus scents can help deceive our brain into thinking that our stomachs are full and therefore stopping that tummy from sending hungry signals to the brain.

The citrus family is a huge one. Citrus fruits have always benefited mankind in many ways. In this chapter, we will highlight the weight loss benefits of using essential oils from these zesty treats. The following items contain the basic aromatherapy profiles of four of the most common citrus fruits that are used as essential oils. And among the other citrus essential oils, they have been found to have the most profound effect for helping with weight loss issues. Also included in the following is additional information on each of these citrus fruits, like their uses in both medical and practical purposes since the early times.

ORANGE.

First up is this iconic orange-colored fruit. Different types of orange peels can yield their essential oils through the process of cold expression. Essential oils from oranges are the most commonly added ingredients to various beauty products.

Anti-aging creams, energizing body lotions, refreshing body wash variants, and other body care products use orange essential oils. Likewise, household items such as scented candles, aerosol deodorizing sprays, and other scented products use orange essential oils.

Orange essential oils are quite often used in pastries and dishes as a flavoring and you would have ingested it more often than you are aware of. That being said, you might become skeptical as to the efficacy of it, since you have never directly felt any of its supposed properties in aiding you to lose weight and control your appetite.

The main reason for this is that the amount you absorb is not enough for you to be able to feel the supposed effects. It can only act as a mood booster but that is pretty much the best you can get out of consuming that much. In order for you to feel the weight loss benefits, the orange essential oil must be in purely organic and undiluted form. That is why it is important to buy the pure concentrated essential oils from trusted sources.

However, you must not confuse the fruit with the oil. The orange fruit is absolutely delicious and refreshing to the taste buds to eat. But the pure, undiluted orange oil is not to be eaten the way you would the fruit. To be able to benefit from the oil, you must use it in an aromatherapy session to help you control your cravings and cope with the everyday stress you encounter that leads you to overeat.

Many health benefits are also attributed to this essential oil because of its properties. Orange in its extracted form is an antidepressant, anti-inflammatory, antiseptic, antispasmodic, carminative, diuretic, aphrodisiac, and sedative substance. It can also maintain healthy skin and treat acne and dermatitis. Being one of the citrus oils, orange essential oil blends well with others like cloves, cinnamon, ginger, frankincense, sandal wood, and black pepper.

You can put the orange essential oil in a diffuser to fill the room with a lingering, pleasant scent that everyone can savor with you. If you are out and about, you can also bring a portable diffuser or inhaler so you can steadily inhale the refreshing scent of oranges for about five minutes to curb your cravings anytime you get them. You can also use this as a topical treatment. Be warned though that like all citrus, this essential oil has a photo-toxic quality. Try to avoid being under direct sunlight a few hours after application. And remember to test your skin sensitivity towards the oil before actual use.

GRAPEFRUIT.

The next one in line among the citrus family is the grapefruit. Grapefruit essential oils can stop your body from retaining water, which is one of the main causes of bloating, and this can also dissolve fat in the body. The essential oil accomplishes this by releasing the stored fat into the bloodstream so your body can dissolve, absorb, and turn it into energy, helping you feel energized. So you can say goodbye to your cellulites and say hello to toned thighs and arms.

Like orange, grapefruit essential oils can also be a strong suppressant for your cravings. It can help you feel fuller for longer. You can put a few drops of the grapefruit essential oil into your diffuser or inhaler to stop any hunger pangs from making you reach for that bag of chips. Another way is to put a drop of the essential oil in 8 ounces of drinking water to drink before your lunch or dinner. This will stop you from eating more than you should.

Grapefruit essential oils also help uplift your thoughts and moods. Improved moods can help you deal with stress better and help you have a better acceptance of yourself and your body. This can save you from developing any eating disorders, be it eating too much or too little.

You can mix different essentials oils to achieve better results. When you encounter extra stressful days that make you want to dive into a tub of vanilla ice cream, why not dive into your bath tub instead? Try mixing about eight drops of grapefruit essential oil and five drops of ginger essential oil to about two ounces of olive or sweet almond oil in your bath water and soak away to a refreshing relaxation.

The different essential oils you can mix together to relieve stress are lemon, chamomile, lavender, grapefruit, and jasmine essential oils. These essential oils have a calming effect. If you are depressed, uplifting and mood-boosting mixes can be of rose, sandalwood, orange, lavender, grapefruit, and jasmine essential oils. If you are feeling anxious, you can arrange for a massage and add a mixture or bergamot, sandalwood, rose, and lavender to your massage oil or as an incense to chase your anxieties away. Grapefruit essential oil blends best with aromas such as frankincense, bergamot, lavender, and geranium.

Try to avoid this essential oil if you are pregnant and you should check your skin sensitivity for this aroma. Avoid strong sunlight after application which is applicable to all citrus essential oils.

LEMON.

Lemons are popular as a citrus fruit and are commonly used for culinary purposes. It is a good source of vitamins and it naturally aids in digestion. It also has a pleasing and refreshing aroma that adds to the attractiveness of food. They are healthy, delicious and inexpensive. Lemons are found to have properties that they are now valued for, such as being a good antidepressant, antiseptic, antioxidant, astringent, and tonic.

Lemon essential oil is extracted from lemon rinds using cold press. It requires about 3,000 lemons to make a kilo of lemon essential oil. This makes the oils very pure and very potent. It gently detoxifies the body and relieves the body of some intestinal parasites that contribute to ill digestive health. Lemon has the ability to cleanse the body from toxins because of the antioxidant limonene. It works on the immune, respiratory and digestive system to help with healthy function.

Lemon is a great all-rounder for skin and hair care. It makes your hair shiny and your skin increase in luster. It also disinfects and rejuvenates your skin. Lemon oil is also used in dealing with excessively oily skin and dandruff. You can add a drop of lemon essential oil in a glass of water for a refreshing and uplifting drink. Adding lemon oil to your drinking water will also provide you with a refreshing purified drink that can really hydrate you and remove tiredness. It would be a great addition to your water bottled during work-out. As with the abovementioned citrus fruits, lemon essential oil shares the same benefits for people wanting to lose weight and control their eating habits. This is because Lemon essential oil can help tame appetite and reduce the chances of overeating. Lemon blends well with other oils like rose, lavender, sandal wood, ylang-ylang, geranium, and tea tree.

Other than that, Lemon essential oil has a lot of uses for aromatherapy. Some example of this is using it as a cleaning agent for metals, as an antiseptic, as grease stains and gum remover. Because of this, lemon is one of the most popular essential oil used in the blends for aromatherapy. Like all citrus oils, you have to avoid direct sunlight for at least half a day when using this oil because it can cause irritation and allergic reactions. Always test for your skin sensitivity towards the essential oil before initiating use. You can dilute it with carrier oils.

BERGAMOT.

Bergamot is about the size of a typical orange but with a yellow rind like a lemon's. It is also used in many medicinal concoctions. Its benefits are attributed to the plant's properties that include being a deodorant, antibiotic, vulnerary, antispasmodic, antiseptic, analgesic, sedative, disinfectant, antidepressant, and digestive tonic. Bergamot essential oil is strongly sedative and is therefore calming. It is best to use when you are stressed or tense that you want to reach for something decadent. So instead of letting sweets and simple sugars calm your nerves, let bergamot essential oils work for you. You will get the same calming effect without any added calories to your diet. It is also a great aroma to help with your self-image as it offers wellness of one's sense of self.

The oils are extracted from the rind. It has a powerful aroma that is widely used in perfumes as a top-note. Unlike most oils, the bergamot essential oil is derived through the cold compression process. It is commonly added into black tea to create what we know as the Earl Grey tea.

When paired with lavender essential oils, the calming or sedative effect will be more powerful. You can take a clean cloth and put a few drops of bergamot on it then steadily inhale it to help you relax when you are stressed out or when you get the urge to eat when you know you shouldn't. You can also dilute a drop of the oil in a teaspoon of honey and take it as you would cough syrup. You can also make a calming yet delicious drink by diluting a drop of the oil in a small glass of almond or soy milk.

Bergamot blends well with other essential oils that include frankincense, clary sage, jasmine, mandarin, cypress, black pepper, nutmeg, geranium, orange, sandal wood, rosemary, and ylang-ylang. It beautifully complements the other citrus oils used in weight loss aroma therapy so expect a nice scent in your blend.

A warning though is that this oil has to be protected from direct sunlight. It actually becomes poisonous when exposed to the sun. Use a dark bottle for your bergamot essential oil. Keep your bottles in dark, cool storage. After the initial skin sensitivity test when contemplating a use of a new essential oil, you still have to be careful in using this. It is because since it is one of the citrus oils, it makes you photo-sensitive and exposure to direct sunlight after application should be avoided.

Well, now that you are acquainted with the citrus family, let us now get to know the other essential oils that will become your best friends in your war against cellulites.

Chapter 4: Non-citrus Essential Oils

In this chapter, we are going to talk about the not-so-citrus essential oils and how they can help us in expelling adipose tissues that are overstaying in our bodies. The citrus oils focus on boosting metabolism and increasing energy, but many other essential oils, especially those coming from herbs, spices and flowers have proven to exhibit the same characteristics with other health benefits. And while the citruses excite your person just as your mood, these non-citrus aromas bring in relaxation and feelings of wellness.

Herbs and spices have been featured in traditional medicine since time immemorial. Not discounting their general usefulness in the kitchen as a part of any cooking utility. They are included in many Western and Oriental cuisine for their ability to enhance and highlight the food's flavors. But to the rest of humanity, they are quite the preserver and restoratives. The have potent properties that bring about wellness to both the mind and the body. Their aroma has a holistic quality of being both medicine and food for the soul. If your citrus essential oils are best utilized during your work-out sessions and before, during and after meals, herb and spice essential oils are great to have all over your home and for your "me times".

PEPPERMINT.

It is a plant native to Europe that is a cross between spearmint and water mint. Peppermint health benefits include its ability to help respiratory problems, indigestion, fever, nausea, headache, digestive spasms, and it is also a pain reliever. And unlike many other essential oils, the health benefits of peppermint and its oil are already studied and proven scientifically. In fact, there are already peppermint essential oil capsules available that is prescribed by doctors of both modern and alternative medicine.

There is a part of your brain that tells you that your stomach is now filled with your mother's special meatloaf and that it can't accommodate anymore. But sometimes, or should I say most of the time, we ignore what our brain tells us and listen to our eyes and taste buds telling us to eat more. Peppermint specifically works on that part of your brain to make it keep telling you that you are indeed full.

In addition, your tummy will love peppermint because it has proven itself as a great helper for digestion. It resolves a wide variety of digestive ailments. It can help you out if you are having problems with candida, as the condition is often a big influence in losing or gaining weight. Moreover, when you are under heavy emotions like depression or anxiety, it can uplift and lighten your mood and motivate you to be more optimistic. Most importantly, peppermint tastes amazing and will let you give a minty fresh kiss to your special someone.

Before you eat anything, put a couple of drops of peppermint essential oil on a clean cloth or a cotton pad and steadily breathe in vapors. You can also put the drops in a diffuser and inhale your way to a reduced appetite. Likewise, you can put a drop of the peppermint oil in a glass of water for a refreshing drink before each meal. You can also pair it with lemon to get the most energizing and waistline-reducing effect.

This essential oil blends well with other aromas like rosemary, eucalyptus, marjoram and lemon. Using too much peppermint essential oil can result to headaches, heartburn and allergic reactions. Conduct a skin sensitivity test to know exactly if you're sensitive to it. Dilute accordingly per application. The safety measures that apply to any alternative medicine and supplements as well as dietary changes should be sufficient to help manage risks.

SANDALWOOD.

This essential oil is extracted through steam distillation of wood from mature trees. The older the tree, the more oil and the stronger aroma it has. And as to this, Indian Sandalwood is currently the top quality produce since they are on the verge of extinction. That also means that they are very expensive. The Hawaiian variety is also quite expensive. But the Australian variety doesn't show much of the benefits associated with the tree. The most commonly available variant though is the Australian Sandalwood. The health benefits attributed to sandalwood is from its properties that include it being a good antiseptic, antispasmodic, anti-inflammatory, emollient, expectorant, memory booster, hypotensive, tonic and sedative substance.

Sandalwood essential oils also have calming sedative properties that can help you control your eating habits when you are undergoing stressful situations. It helps you combat negative feelings and actions. The feeling of having conquered negativity will relieve you of the stress you were having and so also relieving you the impulse to eat something comforting like you beloved mother's macaroni and cheese.

Sandalwood essential oils may be used with a diffuser to constantly inhale the vapors. You can also dilute a drop of the sandalwood oil in a drop of extra virgin olive oil and then apply it directly on your feet or stomach for faster absorption. You can also take it like you would any medical syrup by adding a drop of sandalwood essential oil to a teaspoon of honey. You can make a delicious drink by mixing a drop of the sandalwood oil to a small glass of rice milk. It is good for soothing the nervous, circulatory and digestive systems and helps their function as a health tonic.

Its other uses are tested through the centuries. It has always been used in medicines, industrial products as well as in skin and beauty treatments. It blends well with essential oils like black pepper, bergamot, lavender, geranium, rose, myrrh and ylang-ylang. When using it as a topical treatment, avoid using it for raw skin and remember to always dilute it with carrier oils. You can use either virgin olive oil or coconut oil.

GINGER.

Originating from India, this is commonly used as a spice. The lowly ginger is quite famous in Asian cuisine for being tummy-friendly. It is this spicy yet mildly sweet ingredient that makes Asian dishes taste really good. But its being tummy-friendly is not just because it makes dishes taste awesome. It is also included in almost all meat dishes because it softens the meat and makes it easier to digest. Both the spice and the oil are used as a flavoring agent and preservative. It is loved by your stomach because of its anti-inflammatory and anti-bacterial properties that makes it healthy and in tip-top shape.

Its health benefits are attributed to the ginger's properties that are actually from the compound Gingerol that gives the spice its pungent hot taste. This spice is known as an antiseptic, carminative, digestive, expectorant, analgesic, aphrodisiac and anti-inflammatory substance. In addition, ginger also has a warming effect on the body because of its being mildly spicy that simulates the body, especially the nervous system. Ginger essential oil has been dubbed as the "oil of empowerment" as it gives off a mild heat that enhances our inner strength, energizing and empowering the body and the mind.

To get the full benefit of ginger essential oil, you can put a couple of drops in a diffuser and inhale the vapors as you would any other essential oils that we have already discussed. You can also apply it directly to your skin or by diluting it first in coconut oil if you have sensitive skin. You can do a skin test first by applying it to your forearm to see if you are sensitive to it or not. If you're using it for aromatherapy, ginger essential oil blends nicely with others that include cedar wood, lemon, eucalyptus, lime, geranium, frankincense, sandalwood, rosemary, myrtle, rosewood, bergamot, orange, and ylang-ylang.

CINNAMON.

Popularly used as a flavoring, this herb originated in Asia, but the shrub is now grown in most tropical places in the world. Its bark is its most important part, having the most uses. Because of allergic reactions to its potent oil, most people choose to use the cinnamon directly instead. Its health benefits are attributed to its properties that include being antifungal, antibacterial, astringent, antimicrobial, and anticlotting.

Cinnamon is known to increase the weight loss effectiveness of all the other essential oils you have read about in this book. Diabetics can find comfort in knowing that cinnamon has been discovered to trigger healthy levels of insulin in the body. It also improves digestion and blood circulation. Its antioxidant properties help in gently detoxifying the body and stimulating the immune system to get to fight against invaders that try to give us colds and flu.

Cinnamon essential oils taken from the leaves and twigs through steam distillation have a mildly spicy and musky scent. Cinnamon is great in aromatherapy. However, cinnamon oil from the bark is not usually used in aromatherapy. Much like ginger essential oils, cinnamon essential oils are also mildly spicy and so it warms up the body as well and fights against exhaustion and depression by empowering the body.

In aromatherapy, you can put a few drops of the cinnamon essential oil in burners or vaporizers to be inhaled steadily to calm you and take your mind off eating out your stress. You can also dilute the oil in your bath water as you soak all your worries away. In addition, you can also simultaneously fight off any outwardly infections while soaking in your cinnamon infused bath water because of the cinnamon oil's antiseptic properties. It blends well with other essential oils used in aromatherapy like rosemary, lemon, cardamom, lavender, and geranium.

Being strongly potent in its pure form, it is not recommended to ingest cinnamon essential oil. It is also required that the concentrate be diluted with a carrier oil when applied topically. Diffusion should also be done with caution as your nasal passages may be irritated with a too strong blend. Check your skin's level of sensitivity to this substance. Avoid applying it, diluted or not, to your face and other sensitive areas. And it's definitely must not be used for children under six years of age.

ROSEMARY.

This herb essential oil is famous for promoting clarity of mind and to help with mental focus and memory. In Ancient Greece, students are actually encouraged to tie Rosemary sprigs and flowers into their hair as they study to improved their insight and retention. But through centuries, many other uses including that in helping weight loss is found for the rosemary essential oil. It is a great antioxidant and also helps in managing cellulite. Amazingly, you can also use this oil to aid in treating constipation and diabetes. Rosemary essential oil is also a part of many scent blends that are made for detoxification.

Rosemary essential oil is taken from the flowering plant through steam distillation. It was widely known as a culinary herb. Many dishes are made with its oil and freshly-gathered leaves. Although the distillation takes both the leaves and the blooms, it is mostly taken from the leaves. The flowers are very delicate and doesn't provide as much oil as its leaves does. It has a very welcoming scent that is used in many combinations with other commonly used essential oils. Rosemary blends well with basil, peppermint, frankincense, clary sage, lavender, cedar wood, lemongrass, thyme, elemi, citronella, chamomile, geranium and cardamom. This herb essential oil is valued for its ability to strengthen the entire body and helps to heal some of the most delicate organs such as the brain, liver and heart.

Traditionally, rosemary oils have been used topically and aromatically. You can use a diffuser to enjoy the mind-opening scent in your home. Sometimes, it is also used as a massage and topical oil especially for treating abdominal pains. You can also place a few drops on your handkerchief so you can have a ready indirect inhaler. But if you have an actual inhaler for your aromatherapy blends, then that's fine as well or you can just bring your bottle and take a tiny little sniff from the top when you require. Many have proven that a mixture of rosemary essential oil and water sprayed in a room and on objects can help remove unwanted odors.

Some people are not used to rosemary, however, since it was volatile in nature. Unless it is prescribed, use the oils as an aroma. If you're going to use it directly on the skin you must test for skin sensitivity before actual use. This scent should be avoided during pregnancy and by people with high blood pressure and epilepsy.

BASIL.

The leaves and seeds of basil are commonly used in cuisines from many parts of the world. The oil is used in many culinary purposes such as the Italian pesto. You'd probably seen the plant in pasta and salads. It is a good source of calcium, magnesium, potassium, vitamin A and iron. This herb is widely used in old times for various medical purposes like treating diarrhea, indigestion, constipation, cough and some skin diseases. Basil essential oil is often used as an effective digestive tonic. It has carminative properties that will provide immediate relief in the stomach and intestines.

Clearing out toxins from the digestive track, basil essential oil helps with the process of losing weight. Other than balancing out irregularities in the digestive track, this herb is also great for improving the luster of dulled skin and hair. Many cosmetic supplements have basil essential oils for toning the skin and treating the symptoms of acne and other skin infections. This is because basil also has an antibacterial property. It is also an analgesic and provides pain relief. When used properly, it can also be applied to quickly relieve bloodshot eyes.

The leaves of the herb are steam-distilled to produce one of the most potent essential oils in aromatherapy. The leaves are featured in many treatments and remedies, but the oils taken from the leaves, stems and flowers have potency greater than that from dried or even fresh leaves. It is blended with some of the most popular oils in treatments. It combines well with lemon, bergamot, rosemary, lime, clary sage, geranium, hyssop, clove bud, juniper, marjoram, eucalyptus, and lavender.

Basil is used aromatically by diffusing or inhaling. It is also used with or without carrier oils for massage and topical treatment. It can also be inhaled from the bottle or a drop rubbed between the hands and cupped over the nose and mouth with natural breathing for several minutes to combat nervousness. You can also use a steam tent, inhaling the basil aroma from it or add a drop in water for an instant mouth rinse.

Dubbed to be the essential oil of "renewal", it has shown benefits that are proven in scientific testing. It is also found to be a mild antioxidant for bronchitis when blended with eucalyptus, fir and rosemary. Using it topically would require testing it for your skin sensitivity first. If the pure oil is too strong for you, dilute it to suit your skin sensitivity. If you are pregnant, avoid the pure oils for a while, sticking to using basil leaves in cooking instead. It shouldn't be used for people with epilepsy. It is better to be safe than sorry after all. Other than that, basil essential oil is practically an all-rounder when it comes to general health and wellness.

Chapter 5: Notes and Reminders on Aromatherapy

Before you go on and read about the recipes and procedures specific to aromatherapy meant to lose weight, you have to first have an organized basic knowledge on the procedures and applications used in aromatherapy. The definition and other explanation as to the function of the treatment are already discussed in the previous chapters. So before you are presented with definite steps to follow in your treatment, be familiar with the general approaches that your therapy might take.

First things first, you need to understand some things about this entire affair. You might have noticed it already in passing, but it's nicer to put things as simply as possible, right?

- The use of essential oils particularly for weight loss is not a cure-all. It is only a part of your weight loss regimen, not the entire thing.

- Just because this treatment can help with your stress and overeating does not mean you can tire yourself out and maintain your previous lifestyle. Avoid temptation and manage your affairs to reduce things that give you stress.

- Equal the passive aromatherapy with active initiative. Eat healthy and exercise.

- You might have started this therapy on a whim, but don't give up just because results seem slow in showing. Just like in any endeavor, keep your determination. For this one, it's more like, let it become part of your habits and normal life.

- Before starting this therapy meant for losing weight that is gained through inactivity and overeating, check if your condition is caused by another reason besides those two. If so, you should look into treating that first before trying this one out.

Now you've gone through that, next up is to know the common applications of essential oils. Note that not all the oils can be used in all the applications. That is why knowing the Essential Oil Profile of the aroma you're interested in should help in dealing with any risk involved, as well as a guide to its proper usage. There are basically three applications, but there are various ways to use the essential oils within each application. The three are: Aromatic, Topical, and Internal.

1. **Aromatic Application**

    This is the most popular application for essential oils. Even regular people not going for aromatherapy treatments know that these oils are great for deodorizing and even appending the scents around the home. But as you now know that there is more to these concentrates than just smelling good. This is because the aroma that is scented is in actuality a fine mist or vapor of the oil that is suspended in the air. Thus it has all the properties and compounds found in the oil and the source, including its health benefits. It is because of this effect on the sense of smell and then to the brain that aromatherapy is very effective in affecting the psychological and physical systems of your body. This would probably the safest approach to aromatherapy, but just the same, pay attention to how your body reacts to the scents. Some of the popular ways to use essential oils aromatically are as follows:

- Direct Inhalation

  You can do this by directly smelling from the bottle, ensuring that your nose is a few inches away from the open top. Or you can also place a drop on your palms, rub them together and cup it on your face like an hospital mask. Inhale the vapors for a few minutes in this case.

- Diffusing

  This is preferable for essential oils that have their effects fade with the application of heat. Also, this also makes the vapors stay in the air for a few hours longer than if you had used potpourri.

- Hot Water Vapor

  Place 1-3 drops of the oil into a pot of boiling water and placing your face near the opening, inhale the steam, covering both your head and the pot with a towel.

- Indirect Inhalation

  Use a cotton ball, your handkerchief, fabric squares, your clothes, your linen and other fabrics you will be in contact with. Place and rub in a few drops of the essential oils on these and inhale them whenever you can.

- Fan, Vent and the like

  Dropping some essential oil to a cloth, place it on the fan frame, on the vents or any air-supply opening. You can do this in your vehicle's air conditioning vents.

- Humidifier

  Cool air humidifiers are considered best for this purpose. Note though, that essential oils can damage plastic over time so choose containers that are made especially for essential oils. Either do this or choose glass-type humidifiers.

- Room Deodorizer

  Combine half a cup of distilled water, half a cup of alcohol like vodka and about 30 drops of your favorite scent in a pretty little jar. Add around 10 bamboo skewers like the ones for barbecues and place them in the bottle such that they stick halfway out.

- Deodorant, Perfume and Cologne

  Dab a drop or two on your pulse points or add 10-15 drops to a teaspoon of water, plus 20-30 drops of vodka to make a cologne or body mist. If you're going to use it as a deodorant, add 3-4 drops to a tablespoon of your favorite carrier oil.

2. Topical Application

This application is still simple, but it would take a little more caution. Although most essential oils can be used in this application, the way they are used differ from oil to oil. Some require precautions and even some of those that aren't can still affect some sensitive skin types with allergic reaction if not used the right way. A must for topical application is a patch testing. Know exactly your skin type and how the oils could affect you. If you have normal skin, the regular precautions are enough. If you have sensitive skin, always dilute your oils for topical use, for this, use a drop of the essential oil for every 1-4 ounces of your carrier oil. There are some oils that will require dilution to avoid irritation no matter what your skin type is because of their potency.

- Massage

  This can be very relaxing and enjoyable way to apply essential oils. This is actually one of the more popular uses of the essential oils. Some of the oils can be directly used in a massage, but it is recommended to use carrier oil instead. Not only it will increase the volume of your oils, it would also dilute the mixture to make it safe for topical application. Not all essential oils are safe for this use though. Always check what type of essential oil you are using and if its recommended applications match your intended purpose.

- Hot or Cold Compresses

  The water used for soaking your compresses would have a few drops on it. For the hot compress, a towel soaked in your water-oil mixture and wrapped around a hot water bottle will work.

- Reflexology

  Massaging the oils directly on reflex points associated to your concern. These points are found all over the body, but for this purpose, those in the hands, feet and ears are most preferred.

- Baths

  Add the oils to your bathwater, to your body wash, in your bath salts, or even directly on your wash cloths.

- Personal Care

  You can add a few drops to carrier oil as deodorant. You can also choose to add a few drops into your body effects like lotions, moisturizers and such.

3. **Internal Application**

This application is to be regarded with utmost care. That is because most essential oil providers will have notes that will tell you whether or not your chosen oil can be ingested and used internally. If it safe to do so, here are popular ways to do it:

- Drinking

  Beverages that are usually used are rice milk, almond milk, or water. Lemon combined with peppermint or separately used on your favorite drinks is great for digestion, exhaustion, energy and metabolism.

- Cooking

  Many essential oils are used this way. Just observe the proper way of doing so. Many recipes feature essential oils that can enhance the food's taste and increase nutritional and health benefits.

- Supplemental

  Add a drop to a teaspoon of honey to be taken as a supplement. There are also ready-made supplement oils blend capsules sold in stores or you can make your own by purchasing empty capsules. But remember that you can't store home-filled capsules because the essential oils will dissolve them right after.

- Suppositories and Inserts

  It is very important that you are already using the essential oils and that you know that you are not sensitive to it before you consider this use. Anal suppositories and inserts as well as vaginal inserts are more direct ways of getting the oils into the area of concern. The use of anal or vaginal syringe is more common although there are more comfortable ways to do them. For vaginal inserts, you can soak up the diluted oil mixture into a tampon and use that. And for anal inserts, you can place the mixture into an empty capsule and use it as a suppository. This way the oil is retained in the body for longer periods.

Now you have the basics down pat, what follows would be to try out a few recipes that are proven effective in enhancing energy, metabolism and self-approval and induce weight loss. You can easily find out a concoction that is perfect for you, but here are a few recipes where you can start out. Many have already attested to their efficacy, so read on!

Another thing, for getting your first batch of essential oils, you'll find that these suggestions are too many. So to help, you can note the Big Four of weight loss in the world of essential oils:

- Peppermint: this helps suppress cravings, so this is mostly the support oil.

  - Usual use in weight loss: inhale during bouts of food craving and added to warm baths in the morning.

- Bergamot: it reduces your cholesterol levels (major hint: reduce not obliterate), it just tones it down to safer levels.

  - Usual use in weight loss: blended for diffusion.

- Grapefruit: increases metabolism, this one will help you trim the excesses.

- Usual use in weight loss: added to drinking water for an instant refresher.

- Lemon: boosts metabolism (citruses do that) and improves digestion.

  - Usual use in weight loss: added to drinking water for a refreshing and energizing drink. This is also great during work-outs and in hot weather.

One of the more popular recipes though is to blend a mixture of some choice essential oils to make a topical concoction. Here is one specially designed for that twice-a-day abdominal rub.

1. In a mixing cup, measure out two ounces of a carrier oil. You have a choice among sweet almond oil, virgin olive oil or virgin coconut oil.

2. Add 5 drops each of three essential oils to your mixing cup: lemon grapefruit and cypress. Provided you have tested each of the oils for your sensitivity, you can change the combination to your taste. The four mentioned before do blend well and can make quite the scent!

3. Pour into a glass bottle and securing the lid, roll it between your palms. This is how you mix delicate liquids and you might have already rolled test tubes between your palms in chemistry class a time or two.

4. Use the oil as an abdominal rub, once or twice a day depending on your preference. When massaging your tummy, do so in large circles. Begin above your belly button, working outwards and towards the left of your

abdomen. Keep at it daily or at least five days in a week to show results.

5. Safety Note: Try to avoid sunlight for at least three hours after your belly rub. The citrus oils in your blend cause a slight photosensitivity. Although extreme cases are actually rare, discontinue if any redness, rashes or any allergic reaction appears.

Now on to the other essential oil pin-ups for weight loss:

- Although citrus essential oils are the most popular appetite-curbing oils out there, some people are not too fond of their scent. And cats rather avoid citrus scents. But you have other choices as well that might pique your aroma preference and still satiate your cravings without indulging in comfort foods. Here are a few that are also effective in fighting off that cravings attack:

  - Cumin: usually for cooking

  - Clary Sage: also great for insomnia and hormone balancing

  - Fennel: this is usually used to increase lactation, and to treat blood clotting as well as digestive issues

  - Dill: popular for helping with treatments for gas, constipation, colic and cholesterol problems

  - Ginger: used for vertigo, digestive issues and low libido

- Patchouli: popular for skin issues, insect bites and works as an insect repellant

- Sandalwood: there are so many uses for it, it's among the most-used essential oils for all time

- Peppermint: great for cooking, allergies and digestion

- Vanilla: one of the all-time favorite scents of humanity

- Spearmint: if you want a minty, cool scent

- Ylang-ylang: heady and flowery scent that is pleasant and relaxing

To make these essential oils work to ease your cravings, you have to inhale them for five minutes. Lower than that and you might find your appetite stimulated instead! Most people just carry the bottle with them and inhale a few inches away from the unscrewed top when their appetite spike or when their craving strike. But if the scent becomes too strong for you, consider placing a drop in one palm, rubbing it to the other. Then cup both palms to cover your nose and mouth, inhaling the appetite-suppressing aroma for those five minutes.

- You can make little batches of your own home-made weight loss aromatherapy inhaler. Making it in little batches will enable you to make more. Say, you have one to be carried around in your pack, one in the kitchen, one in your work area, and so on. You can place these where you can easily reach them when the urge to overeat or eat in between meals comes. Not only will it help you quickly quench your cravings, it would also ensure that you are getting your daily dose of weight loss "treatment". You can choose your preferred scent blend from the following list. Or you can circulate through the different blends so you won't get bored from having the same scent day after day. Incidentally, some studies show that this weight loss aromatherapy works more effectively when the scent is changed daily. So it might be a good idea to make a schedule of your scent-for-the-day. Note that all these are blends meant to help with your weight loss regimen so you can actually start with these three in rotation.

- Herbal Blend: when you prefer a spicy aroma.

  - 1 drop Thyme

  - 15 drops Marjoram

  - 1 drop Oregano

  - 15 drops Basil

- Minty Blend: for those times that you want a refreshing scent.

  - 1 drop Ylang-ylang

  - 10 drops Bergamot

  - 4 drops Spearmint

  - 20 drops Peppermint

- Citrus Blend: when you need a zesty, fruity

scent.

- 1 drop Ylang-ylang

- 4 drops Lemon

- 30 drops Grapefruit

In each blend, place a teaspoon of course sea salt in a small dark colored glass bottle and place the oils in drop by drop. Then as mentioned before, blend it by rolling the bottle between your palms. You have to make sure that the essential oils that you use for these are pure and of good quality. Sometimes you have to test out different vendors to find your preferred price and quality. And by then, you can sense minute differences between their scents, which are usually an indicator of quality. This can make you prefer a seller than the others.

Use these blends when your appetite spikes and before eating. The more often you inhale your weight loss aromatherapy, the more effective it will be. To use your inhaler, take three slow and long deep breaths of the day's aroma blend. Take a break, since you don't want to hurt your sinuses, right? Then do it again. Do this procedure three times, until you've flooded your sense with the aroma, having taken nine lungful breaths of the blend.

- Now you have quite some ways to deal with the physical aspect of your "food addiction". It is also quite useful to consider the emotional and psychological aspect of the problem, right? After all, weight problems are also caused or aggravated by negative emotional climates. It also causes really negative feelings that will impede with your treatment. Also, there are instances that it is your emotions that trigger your cravings.

- Vanilla essential oil can help you feel secure, comfortable and at home. Its familiar sweet scent will help you resist that cookie.

- Chocolate essence has a rich, sweet scent that can replace that chocolate craving.

- Chamomile has a gentle, flowery scent that will help you relax that stressed mind that makes you want to binge.

- Rose will help with your self-image, giving you confidence in your own skin, owing to its mild aphrodisiac effect.

- Ylang-ylang has been mentioned in the past recipes, as it helps with your self-love which is important in any lifestyle change therapy.

Chapter 6: A Helper and Complement

These essential oils that we have discussed in this book will only be effective if you work hard at your goal as well. Remember that nothing can replace proper diet and regular exercise to help you keep fit and healthy. But these essential oils can greatly help you in your struggle in picking up that mouth-watering sandwich and take a bite off of it when you are not genuinely hungry.

These previously mentioned essential oils will boost you the two other main weapons in your war against excess fat. They have the properties that will let your body break down those stored reserves and turn them to energy. They help in controlling your appetite and sudden cravings. Finally, they affect certain parts of the brain that will calm you and help you relax. This part is important because although you don't notice it, a major reason for overeating is excessive stress and anxieties.

Of course, disciplining yourself to eat the right kinds of food and to have a regular exercise program is difficult at first. You might be dreading having to eat only healthy food or having to go to the gym or even just increasing your daily physical activity. It might be the very reason that you have bought this book, trying to find a way to lose weight without having to follow a proper diet and a regular exercise plan.

Well, following the instructions above and using essential oils alone in your goal of losing weight is indeed a possibility. It is not impossible. Many busy individuals who chose to follow these instructions have succeeded in steadily losing weight over time. But it is definitely slower and only because they were truly busy in their life in the meanwhile. However, for the most cases, it is usually not enough and more so if you continue to live a sedentary lifestyle and choose unhealthy kinds of food. There should be balance in everything. One way or another, you are going to have to face the consequences of your actions, or rather your inaction. Also following the same logic, mustering up your will power to deal with this now with all your determination will earn you amazing rewards later on. Thus, the choice still rests in you.

It is not at all daunting to follow a proper diet plan and a regular exercise program. But first, you have to want to make yourself healthier. Without your will and motivation, you most probably will not succeed. Moreover, you need to be consistent and steady with your routine to reach your goal of losing weight and keeping fit. If you are not consistent, you will undergo a yo-yo pattern, in which you will lose weight when you are motivated and gain weight when you are not.

It is not only bad for your health, it is also bad for your physical appearance as well because a yo-yo diet will ruin the elasticity of your skin causing it to have stretch marks and that will not be a very nice sight to see. Losing weight gradually coupled with good exercise will give your skin the time to adjust and fit your new size, reducing the possibility of stretch marks and skin flaps that are commonly seen in people undergoing crash diets. And that is another reason why this aromatherapy combined with a regular, albeit healthier, diet and light exercise is preferable than many three-week over-correction methods. These are those methods where you push your limits for a short period of time to pull your body status to nearly zero and then adjusting to a healthier normal diet from there. People who have tried those crash diets and suffered setbacks from it as well as those who didn't want to end up suffering like so would actually find this book's instructions quite enjoyable.

The food you eat also plays a big role in your goal to losing weight. Aside from keeping your body healthy in general, vitamins in fruits and vegetables, particularly vitamins A and E, will greatly increase your skins elasticity and give you a rosy glow on your cheeks suggesting you are indeed in the "pink of health". Unlike over-correction methods, you do not need to cut out of your regular meals. You're just going to have to trim the snack-times away by quenching your appetite when the urge to eat appears. You can still eat the same food, but you now have a chance to think through your raging appetite and choose how much you will eat. It would also make deciding on healthier choices easier.

Some of the essential oils mentioned in this book will enable you to keep up a regular routine of exercise and physical activity. Orange and peppermint essential oils will perk you up and keep you feeling energized and motivated to follow your exercise program. Having them combined into the drinking water you bottle for working out can give you an additional boost whenever you feel your energy slacken. Cinnamon and ginger essential oils will empower you to keep going even when you feel like you can't go on anymore.

Sandalwood and bergamot essential oils will calm and relax your nerves when you are feeling stressed out so you can win against the temptations of rich desserts and deep fried foods. And the best part about these essential oils is that it gives no side effects as it is completely natural and pure, having no caffeine, no sugar, and no preservatives.

A word of caution though: you may find some shops selling

essential oils, usually containing a mixture of grapefruit, coconut, cedar, and other essential oils, claiming to burn fat. It would be great for calming and energizing you as discussed above. However, these cannot really help you to break down fat or cellulite in your body. It may temporarily make your skin look firmer because it hydrates your skin, but it is not a permanent fix. This is the reason why you are presented in the previous chapters about what each essential oil do, so you will know exactly what each blend can give you.

It is better to research and experiment about which aromatherapy works best for you. Make sure that you do your homework and that you know how to properly use diffusers or inhalers to get the best out of your essential oils. When applying the essential oils directly on your body, make sure you dilute it first in carrier oil such as virgin olive oil or coconut oil. Remember as well that some essential oils can be toxic to you if you directly ingest it. Always keep them in a safe place away from young children. Unless you have been using the essential oils for some time, only follow specific recipes to make sure it is safe for you. For example, the blends produced by the instructions in the previous chapter are generally safe for use by anyone being as they are made from compatible essential oils. But do remember to test each blend produced whether or not you are sensitive to them as discussed before. You can easily do this by applying the oil on a small part of your skin, you can choose to dilute it or not, and see if any undesirable reaction occurs. Usually the patch test is done on the inside of the wrist, beneath the ear or on the inside of the elbow.

Chapter 7: A Look in the Mirror

A mirror helps you to see yourself to check if you need to adjust your tie, if you need to reapply your lipstick, or if you have a piece of red bell pepper stuck to your teeth. But sometimes people forget to look at their inner mirror to check if the way they think or see things is correct. You need to take a good long look at yourself as well.

You need to honestly ask yourself whether you are doing this for yourself, to make yourself a better and healthier person or whether you are doing this just to please someone else. It is true that you need to present yourself well and make sure you look presentable when dealing with other people. It is one of the best forms of respect after all. But you should not change yourself just to please someone who does not genuinely care about you. You must be absolutely sure that if you choose to do this, you have decided to do so by your own volition and entirely for yourself.

The motivation to lose weight should come from you, not from anyone else. Moreover, you should do it for the right reasons. When you are guided by a proper motivation and you have the right reasons to embark on the journey to weight loss, you will have more stability and consistency all throughout.

That stability will give you a reason to go on even when you encounter setbacks in your goals, such as an unexpected dinner celebration for your friend's promotion or a relapse into pigging out during a family reunion, which ruins your carefully planned out diet. It may also be a surprise added workload, which meant you would have to give up going to the gym for a few days to accommodate the added workload. In such cases you have to have a sort of "make-up" plan to replace the wasted time and to balance out those additional calories. You should have your own version of an income-expense balance sheet, either in your mind or in your journal, if you have one. This will make setting up a goal of expending that income of calories much easier. But sometimes, it is really hard, even then. And when that happens, will power will be your anchor. You should have a solid determination to reach your goals or else, your journey's end will be in danger.

You need to be able to motivate yourself to continue even when setbacks happen. However, you will not always be strong. You should be iron-willed in these times. Having an option of backing out will make you feel as if your weight loss journey is too difficult. Give yourself no choice but to keep n moving and trudging onwards. Moments of weakness can dim one's resolve and make them doubt their own determination. Therefore, having a loved one or a friend know of your goals and asking for their support will greatly help you win the war against your bulges. You can also have a "weight loss buddy" whom you can be with as you journey towards a better health and a better self.

Having someone to exercise and eat proper amounts and right kinds of food with will make exercising and dieting less boring and tiresome. Knowing that you are in this together will empower you more while you let the essential oils work their magic to boost your energy. You can take essential oil-infused baths together or have your massages using your favorite essential oils together. And when "times get hard" and your motivations wane, you can encourage each other and become each other's anchor into the determination to lose those excesses.

You may have to start this journey to a good figure and a better lifestyle alone. But getting and earning support along the way as well as sharing the experience with the people around you can make the results that much more rewarding. You can even find yourself helping another in their own journey towards their better self.

Not only will you be benefited by your regular exercise program, your proper healthy diet, and the essential oils we have discussed in this book, but you will also be benefited by the soothing and calming effect of human connection. All these things add up to make your whole weight loss journey more pleasant. Remember that those are puzzle pieces that need to be put together in order for you to complete the picture.

Chapter 8: Some Inspiration

A major part of the big picture is being at peace with your own self throughout your weight loss journey. That is why the moments when you're enjoying the peace and clarity of mind induced by essential oils should be spent for your self-betterment. Here are a few weight loss inspirational quotes you can contemplate on in your "me" times.

- You should be patient because success is not a race.
  Every little success will lead you to that dream Success.
  That dream Success requires constant work and progress.
  Success isn't something you wait for; you have to go get it.
  You have to focus on the entire process because the journey describes your Success and not the destination.
  Stop dreaming about Success, wake up and start working for it.
  Those who have tried and kept on trying will win and maintain Success.
  What is a good day to Succeed? Every day!
  That good old "if at first you don't then try again and again".
- If you think your progress have slowed down and plateaued, think that it's just a little rest before reaching your goal. Maintaining your goal figure is a long plateau anyway, so why not practice for that?
- Whatever you experience can teach you something. It just depends on how you will see things. Just

remember that success isn't much of a success without experiencing failures.

- Once you make your decision, you have to start doing something, even if it's very small, because without that first tiny step, you won't reach the end line.
- Your past will affect your future, but that doesn't mean your past will be the sole dictator of your future.
- Would it simply be enough to know what to do? Or are you going to get up and do it?
- All ends with this question: What do you want? And how far are you willing to go to get it?
- Empower yourself with specific words of a specific image that you dream for yourself. And then believe in it and in yourself.
- We can heal the damages wrought on our bodies by years of bad habit, it all starts with raising your personal standards and minding what you put in it.
- All things are possible, the question remains whether you're going to do it or not.
- The dictionary can give you what Discipline means. The military can give you a glorious definition for it. But basically? It's just remembering exactly what you want.
- The people, who get up one more time than they fall, make it through.
- Having the determination to not quit today will be your success tomorrow.
- Always remember that quitting is not an option. Because quitters don't win!
- Do what you have to and do what you can. Soon, you'll see yourself doing what you want.

- Your life in the future is just a collation of what you did today ad how you did them.
- Don't sacrifice your goal for something that won't even be in your body a day after.
- Remember that what you wanted the most is not worth losing for something you just wanted for the moment.
- You might not see things change in an instant, but you have to have the patience to reach the day you'll see it.
- The best time is now. Don't hesitate just go. Remove "next time" from your vocabulary, it's so counter-productive.
  As they say, yesterday is a memory, tomorrow is a dream, but today is the reality.
  That's just saying that set goals you can achieve within this 24 hours you have right now.
- Trials become obstacles and difficulties become impossible when you forget what you're aiming for.
- The chances you'll hit your target increase when you raise your arms, think, aim and fire!
- Your thoughts become words, your words become actions. Your actions become habits which in turn become character. Watch your character because it will then become your destiny!
- You can only face a fear when you know its name. And you can only defeat your fear when you face it!
- Worrying about tomorrow wouldn't solve problems still in the future. It would only make your day miserable.
- You must get on with your journey sure of getting to the end.
- Procrastination kills a good idea even before it takes

flight.

- Unless you try something you haven't done yet, you wouldn't learn. And if you don't learn, you won't grow.
- A night road doesn't seem that dark when you look at that bright light at your goal's end.
- When you become content with something less than what you want, you will get even lesser than what you can be content with.
- It is not leaping giant steps that will get you to the end. It is those strong, sure, little steps!
- They always say that when one door, another would open. But oftentimes we stare longingly at that closed door to actually notice that another have opened elsewhere.
- Don't say "I can't do this", ask "How can I do this?"
- You can never win if you're afraid to lose.
- Failure will not kill you. Not trying to change will.
- Successful people are those who realize that their failures are preparing them for their victories.
- If we keep on doing something, despite difficulties, it becomes easier. The thing itself didn't become easy; we just became more able to do it.
- Success is not the finished product; it's just the cherry on top. Success is the process between, usually one where's the only ingredient is to not quit.

Keep the feelings communicated by these words and you'll find yourself reminded of what you want and what goal you have set for yourself, every time. Numerous times, it has already been proven that essential oils combined with active participation and an openness to change can help individuals reach their lifestyle goals. Add some of the right attitudes, and it will be a formula for your weight loss journey's success!

Conclusion

Thank you again for purchasing this book!

I hope this book was able to help you to realize the hidden potential of certain essential oils in weight loss, in increasing your body's energy, in uplifting your mood and countenance, and in improving your overall well-being.

The next step is to apply what you have learned in this book and to get you going on your way to physical fitness and better health. Remember that these facts about the essential oils mentioned above will be useless if you do not work hard and work steady. Avoid the yo-yo and crash diets. Slow and steady wins the race too. And in the race to weight loss, the fast and furious method won't really cut it. Take your time and enjoy your journey to a thinner and more healthy you!

Finally, if you enjoyed this book, please take the time to share your thoughts and post a review on Amazon. We do our best to reach out to readers and provide the best value we can. Your positive review will help us achieve that. It'd be greatly appreciated!

Thank you and good luck!

Check Out My Other Books

Below you'll find some of my other popular books that are popular on Amazon and Kindle as well. Simply click on the links below to check them out. Alternatively, you can visit my author page on Amazon to see other work done by me.

Coconut Oil for Easy Weight Loss: A Step by Step Guide for Using Virgin Coconut Oil for Quick and Easy Weight Loss

http://www.amazon.com/Coconut-Oil-Easy-Weight-Loss-ebook/dp/B00JG8H8DE

Superfoods that Kickstart Your Weight Loss Learn How to Use 30 Superfoods to Boost Weight Loss, Immunity and to Live a Healthier Lifestyle

http://www.amazon.com/Superfoods-that-Kickstart-Your-Weight-ebook/dp/B00JNAPM9M

Carrier Oils for Beginners: Discover the Characteristics and Beauty and Health Benefits of Carrier Oils For mixing Aromatherapy Essential Oils

http://www.amazon.com/Carrier-Oils-Beginners-Characteristics-Aromatherapy-ebook/dp/B00K88GI2S

Natural Homemade Cleaning Recipes For Beginners: Essential Oil Recipes For Household Cleaning, Laundry & Toxic Free Living http://www.amazon.com/Natural-Homemade-Cleaning-Recipes-Beginners-ebook/dp/B00K87UBQI

The Best Secrets of Natural Remedies: The Ultimate Guide to Natural Remedies to Prevent and Cure Illnesses, Cold and Flu for Your Family

http://www.amazon.com/Best-Secrets-Natural-Remedies-Illnesses-ebook/dp/B00JNDCOCM

The Hypothyroidism Handbook:An Everyday Guide to Natural Solutions of living with Hypothyroidism including increased energy, lasting weight loss, and general well-being

http://www.amazon.com/Hypothyroidism-Handbook-Solutions-including-increased-ebook/dp/B00JNIGIV0

The Hyperthyroidism Handbook: An Everyday Guide to Natural Solutions of Living with Hyperthyroidism including Weight Gain, Increased Energy and General Well-being

http://www.amazon.com/Hyperthyroidism-Handbook-Solutions-including-Hypothyroidism-ebook/dp/B00JOHU5SM

Essential Oils & Weight Loss for Beginners: Ultimate Guide to Losing Weight, Increasing Energy, Balancing Metabolism & Appetite Using Essential Oils & Aromatherapy

http://www.amazon.com/Essential-Oils-Weight-Loss-Beginners-ebook/dp/B00JOFOWP6

Top Essential Oil Recipes: A Recipe Guide Of Natural, Non-Toxic Aromatherapy & Essential Oils for Healing Common Ailments, Beauty, Stress & Anxiety http://www.amazon.com/Top-Essential-Oil-Recipes-Aromatherapy-ebook/dp/B00JY434E2

Soap Making For Beginners: A Guide to Making Natural Homemade Soaps from Scratch, Includes Recipes and Step by Step Processes for Making Soaps

http://www.amazon.com/Soap-Making-Beginners-Homemade-Processes-ebook/dp/B00JYKH75I

Body Butters For Beginners: Proven Secrets To Making All Natural Body Butters For Rejuvenating And Hydrating Your Skin

http://www.amazon.com/Body-Butters-Beginners-Rejuvenating-Hydrating-ebook/dp/B00K6LVV6A

Apple Cider Vinegar For Beginners: Proven Secrets Using Apple Cider Vinegar For Health, Weight Loss, and Skin Care

http://www.amazon.com/Apple-Cider-Vinegar-Beginners-Aromatherapy-ebook/dp/B00K6YY6HI

Homemade Body Scrubs & Masks For Beginners: 50 Proven All Natural, Easy Recipes For Body & Facial Masks To Exfoliate Nourish, & Care For Your Skin

http://www.amazon.com/Homemade-Body-Scrubs-Masks-Beginners-ebook/dp/B00K79D4SY

Essential Oils Box Set #1: Essential Oils & Weight Loss For Beginners (Ultimate Guide to Losing Weight, Increasing Energy, Balancing Metabolism & Appetite Using Essential Oils & Aromatherapy) + Top Essential Oil Recipes (A Recipe

Guide of Natural, Non-Toxic Aromatherapy & Essential Oils for Healing Common Ailments, Beauty, Stress & Anxiety)

http://www.amazon.com/ESSENTIAL-OILS-BOX-SET-Aromatherapy-ebook/dp/B00K7Q8HRK

Essential Oils Box Set #2: Essential Oils & Weight Loss For Beginners (Ultimate Guide to Losing Weight, Increasing Energy, Balancing Metabolism & Appetite Using Essential Oils & Aromatherapy) + Top Essential Oil Recipes (A Recipe Guide of Natural, Non-Toxic Aromatherapy & Essential Oils for Healing Common Ailments, Beauty, Stress & Anxiety)

http://www.amazon.com/ESSENTIAL-OILS-BOX-SET-Aromatherapy-ebook/dp/B00K7Q8HRK

Box Set#3: Coconut Oil for Easy Weight Loss(A Step by Step Guide for Using Virgin Coconut Oil for Quick and Easy Weight Loss) + Apple Cider Vinegar(Proven Secrets Using Apple Cider Vinegar for Health, Weight Loss, and Skin Care)

http://www.amazon.com/Box-Set-Beginners-Aromatherapy-Essential-ebook/dp/B00K9TEGUW

Box Set #4: Body butters For Beginners(Proven Secrets To Making All Natural Body Butters For Rejuvenating And Hydrating Your Skin) & Top Essential Oil Recipes: A Recipe Guide Of Natural, Non-Toxic Aromatherapy & Essential Oils for Healing Common Ailments, Beauty, Stress & Anxiety

http://www.amazon.com/Box-Set-Butters-Beginners-Essential-ebook/dp/B00KA02F4Y

Box Set #5: Soap Making For Beginners(A Guide to Making Natural Homemade Soaps from Scratch, Includes Recipes and Step by Step Processes for Making Soaps) + Homemade Body Scrubs & Masks For Beginners(50 Proven All Natural, Easy Recipes For Body Scrub & Facial Masks To Efoliate, Nourish, & Care For Your Skin)

http://www.amazon.com/Box-Set-Beginners-Homemade-Recipes-ebook/dp/B00K9U3I2I

Box Set #6: Body Butters for Beginners (Proven Secrets To Making All Natural Body Butters For Rejuvenating And Hydrating Your Skin) +Homemade Body Scrubs & Masks For Beginners(50 Proven All Natural, Easy Recipes For Body Scrub & Facial Masks To Exfoliate, Nourish, & Care For Your Skin)

http://www.amazon.com/Box-Set-Beginners-Exfoliating-Moisturizing-ebook/dp/B00K9U3Y40

Box Set #7: TOP ESSENTIAL OILS(A Recipe Guide Of Natural, Non-Toxic Aromatherapy & Essential Oils For Healing, Common Ailments, Beauty, Stress & Anxiety) & THE BEST SECRETS OF NATURAL REMEDIES(The Ultimate Guide to Natural Remedies to Prevent and Cure Illnesses, Cold and Flu for Your Family)

http://www.amazon.com/BOX-SET-Essential-Recipes-Remedies-ebook/dp/B00K9WPMQG

Box Set #8: NATURAL HOMEMADE CLEANING RECIPES FOR BEGINNERS (Essential Oil Recipes for Household Cleaning, Laundry & Toxic Free Living) + TOP ESSENTIAL OILS(A Recipe Guide Of Natural, Non-Toxic Aromatherapy & Essential Oils For Healing, Common Ailments, Beauty, Stress & Anxiety)

http://www.amazon.com/BOX-SET-Beginners-Essential-Aromatherapy-ebook/dp/B00KAMNGBS

Box Set #9: Essential Oils & Weight Loss for Beginners (Ultimate Guide to Losing Weight, Increasing Energy, Balancing Metabolism & Appetite Using Essential Oils & Aromatherapy) + Carrier Oils for Beginners (Discover the Characteristics and Beauty and Health Benefits of Carrier Oils for Mixing Aromatherapy Essential Oils)

http://www.amazon.com/BOX-SET-Essential-Beginners-Aromatherapy-ebook/dp/B00KAODL6Q

BOX SET #10: THE HYPERTHYROIDISM HANDBOOK (An Everyday Guide to Natural Solutions of Living with Hyperthyroidism including Weight Gain, Increased Energy and General Well-being) + THE HYPOTHYROIDISM HANDBOOK (Everyday Guide to Natural Solutions of Living With Hypothyroidism Including Increased Energy, Lasting Weight Loss, and General Well-Being)

http://www.amazon.com/BOX-SET-10-Hyperthyroidism-Hypothyroidism-ebook/dp/B00KAKMSBY

BOX SET #11: CARRIER OILS FOR BEGINNERS (Discover the Characteristics and Beauty and Health Benefits of Carrier Oils for Mixing Aromatherapy Essential Oils) + Essential Oils & Aromatherapy for Beginners (Secrets to Beauty, Health and Weight Loss Using Proven Essential Oil and Aromatherapy Recipes

http://www.amazon.com/BOX-SET-Beginners-Essential-Aromatherapy-ebook/dp/B00KAONEQ8

BOX SET 12: ESSENTIAL OILS & WEIGHT LOSS FOR

BEGINNERS: (Ultimate Guide to Losing Weight, Increasing Energy, Balancing Metabolism & Appetite Using Essential Oils & Aromatherapy) + TOP ESSENTIAL OIL RECIPES (A Recipe Guide of Natural, Non-Toxic Aromatherapy & Essential Oils for Healing Common Ailments, Beauty, Stress & Anxiety) + CARRIER OILS FOR BEGINNERS (Discover the Characteristics & Beauty & Health Benefits of Carrier Oils for Mixing Aromatherapy Essential Oils) + ESSENTIAL OILS & AROMATHERAPY FOR BEGINNERS (Secrets to Beauty & weight Loss Using Proven Essential Oil & Aromatherapy Recipes) + NATURAL HOMEMADE CLEANING RECIPES FOR BEGINNERS (Essential Oil Recipes for Household Cleaning, Laundry & Toxic Free Living)

http://www.amazon.com/BOX-SET-12-Essential-Aromatherapy-ebook/dp/B00KCBCHE4

BOX SET #13: SUPERFOODS THAT KICKSTART YOUR WEIGHT LOSS (Learn How to Use 30 Superfoods to Boost Weight Loss, Immunity and to Live a Healthier Lifestyle) + ESSENTIAL OILS & AROMATHERAPY FOR BEGINNERS (Secrets to Beauty, Health and Weight Loss Using Proven Essential Oil and Aromatherapy Recipes) + BODY BUTTERS FOR BEGINNERS (Proven Secrets To Making All Natural Body Butters For Rejuvenating And Hydrating Your Skin) + SOAP MAKING FOR BEGINNERS (A Guide to Making Natural Homemade Soaps from Scratch, Includes Recipes and Step by Step Processes for Making Soaps) + HOMEMADE BODY SCRUBS FOR BEGINNERS (50 Proven All Natural, Easy Recipes For Body Scrub & Facial Masks To Exfoliate, Nourish, & Care For Your Skin)

http://www.amazon.com/BOX-SET-Superfoods-Kickstart-

Aromatherapy-ebook/dp/B00KC8G6DK/

BOX SET 14: Essential Oils & Weight Loss for Beginners (Ultimate Guide to Losing Weight, Increasing Energy, Balancing Metabolism & Appetite Using Essential Oils & Aromatherapy) + Apple Cider Vinegar for Beginners (Proven Secrets Using Apple Cider Vinegar for Health, Weight Loss, and Skin Care) + Body Butters For Beginners (Proven Secrets To Making All Natural Body Butters For Rejuvenating And Hydrating Your Skin)
+ Homemade Body Scrubs & Masks for Beginners (50 Proven All Natural, Easy Recipes for Body Scrub & Facial Masks to Exfoliate, Nourish, & Care for Your Skin) + Coconut Oil for Easy Weight Loss (A Step by Step Guide for Using Virgin Coconut Oil for Quick and Easy Weight Loss)

http://www.amazon.com/BOX-SET-Essential-Beginners-Aromatherapy-ebook/dp/B00KEDO68U

www.ingramcontent.com/pod-product-compliance
Lightning Source LLC
Chambersburg PA
CBHW060222290526
45789CB00003B/1371